Cristiane Marins Ferreira
Regina P. Alvarenga
Carmen Lucia Antão Paiva

Clinical, Radiological and Genetic Investigation of Fahr's Disease

Cristiane Marins Ferreira
Regina P. Alvarenga
Carmen Lucia Antão Paiva

Clinical, Radiological and Genetic Investigation of Fahr's Disease

Clinical Case Study

ScienciaScripts

Imprint

Cover image: www.ingimage.com

This book is a translation from the original published under ISBN 978-613-9-76127-2.

Publisher:
Sciencia Scripts
is a trademark of
Dodo Books Indian Ocean Ltd. and OmniScriptum S.R.L publishing group

120 High Road, East Finchley, London, N2 9ED, United Kingdom
Str. Armeneasca 28/1, office 1, Chisinau MD-2012, Republic of Moldova, Europe
Printed at: see last page
ISBN: 978-620-6-40920-5

DEDICATORY

To everyone, at any age, who is motivated to do science in this country. Let it be an incentive to make a difference.

ACKNOWLEDGEMENTS

To Professor and supervisor Carmen Lúcia Antão Paiva, for her patience and time dedicated to me. Her simplicity made this project easier.

To Prof Regina Maria Papais Alvarenga, eternal teacher and co-supervisor, who made me fall in love with Neurology and always encouraged me to do my Master's degree. The concept of didactics was renewed by her.

To my parents, Walkyr (*in memoriam*) and Iacy, for everything I've achieved so far.

To my dear sister and partner Cristine, soul mate, teacher. Great strength and light on my path.

To Dr Paulo Henrique Godoy, for his long friendship and advice. Your professionalism inspired me.

To the collaborators Dr Cassio Luiz C. Serrão and Dr Suely Rodrigues dos Santos, mutant agents in the evolution of this project.

To Mr Luiz, secretary of Neurology, for finalising the work.

To Felipe Sutter, from CopyArt, for his prompt response to my requests

To the dear Ana Carolina Lopes Abrantes and her family. Without her, none of this would be possible.

To everyone who, in some way, contributed and supported me in the realisation of this achievement.

And finally and above all to the HIGHER BEING, for enlightening my mind and maintaining my inner strength.

SUMMARY

Introduction: Fahr's Disease or Familial Primary Calcification of the Basal Nuclei is a rare, autosomal dominant neurodegenerative disease characterised by symmetrical, bilateral calcifications in the basal nuclei with extrapyramidal and psychiatric symptoms. In recent years, mutations in four genes have been identified as causing the disease (*SLC20A2, PDGFRB, PDGFB* and *XPR1*), allowing for a specific genotype-phenotype correlation. Aim: The aim of this study is to describe clinically and through imaging the case of a patient with Fahr's disease and its appropriate propaedeutics, carrying out a clinical and genetic study on the proband (index case) and on some of her family members, in an attempt to identify whether the affected gene was *SLC20A2*. Methodology: Data was obtained from the proband through clinical examinations. The genetic tests were carried out by geneticist Cássio Luiz Carvalho Serrão. The clinical and genetic data of the proband's family members was obtained by telephone and during anamnesis. Based on this data, the family's heredogram was created using a specific programme (GenoPro). The proband underwent laboratory screening, imaging tests and molecular genetic tests. The *SLC20A2* gene was sequenced by the DLE (Diagnósticos Laboratoriais Especializados) laboratory using DNA extracted from peripheral blood cells. The electroencephalogram showed non-specific alterations. We suggest that exome sequencing be carried out in the future to elucidate the genotype. Results: A white girl presented with her first afebrile seizure at the age of 3. She progressed well until the age of 11 when, in addition to a worsening in the frequency of seizures, she began to show cognitive decline, intense migraine-like headaches and tremors. A CT scan of the skull revealed multiple symmetrical calcifications in the basal nuclei and the family history was positive for genetic disease: the father had seizures since the age of 6, cognitive impairment and a radiological image similar to his daughter. Considering the clinical picture, the progression of the disease, laboratory and imaging tests, the hypothesis of Fahr's disease was considered. The proband and her immediate family members were referred to the Genetics department for specific tests to investigate a mutation in the main candidate gene (*SLC20A2*). Conclusion: Although rare, Fahr's disease should be investigated in patients with movement disorders, seizures and calcifications in the basal ganglia. It is suggested that an evaluation of parents up to the third generation should be carried out. The genetic evaluation of our patient showed no alterations in the *SLC20A2* gene or variations in chromosomes 9 and 22. There are no previous case studies of this disease in the state of Rio de Janeiro.

Keywords: Fahr's syndrome. Fahr's disease. Familial Primary Calcifications of the Basal Glands. Idiopathic Calcifications of the Basal Ganglia. Bilateral striated-pallid-tooth calcinosis.

SUMMARY

CHAPTER 1

INTRODUCTION

Fahr's disease (FD) or Familial Primary Calcification of the Basal Nuclei is a rare neurodegenerative disease, with an incidence of less than 1 per 1 million inhabitants (SALEEM et al., 2013) worldwide, autosomal dominant, characterised by symmetrical and bilateral calcifications in the basal nuclei (nb) and other areas of the cerebral cortex, thus allowing for diverse clinical presentations, mainly with extrapyramidal and psychiatric symptoms. In recent years, mutations in four genes have been identified as causing the disease (*SLC20A2, PDGFRB, PDGFB and XPR1*) allowing for a specific genotype-phenotype correlation as shown in Table 1 (TADIC et al., 2015).

The author is a neurologist working in the field of neuropediatrics. Through clinical history and examinations, she diagnosed the proband with FD and found the means to develop this work in postgraduate studies.

1.1 JUSTIFICATION AND RELEVANCE

Although FD is rare, the diversity of its clinical presentations makes it important in the context of differential diagnosis, when faced with patients with metabolic alterations and other relatives with similar conditions. In these cases, knowing the disease in order to order an accurate genetic study is important in order to make the genotype-phenotype correlation. As well as drawing attention to the possibility of the disease in this context, this work is relevant because, at the time of writing, there were no other descriptions of cases of the disease in the state of Rio de Janeiro, using molecular and radiological tests.

CHAPTER 2

LITERATURE REVIEW

2.1 HISTORY

The first description of the disease was in 1850 by Delacour in France, who first recognised the "ossification" of the cerebral capillary vessels in a 56-year-old patient with weakness, tremor and rigidity of the distal extremities (DELACOUR, 1850).

In 1855, Bamberger described the case of a 56-year-old woman with cognitive decline, calcifications in the cerebral vessels and a seizure (BAMBERGER, 1855).

Finally, in 1930, the German pathologist Karl Theodor Fahr reported the case of an 81-year-old male patient with dementia, immobility without paralysis, seizures, whose anatomopathological examination revealed diffuse calcifications of vessels and basal nuclei (FAHR et al., 1930). He was the first to use the term "idiopathic non-arteriosclerotic cerebral calcification of the cerebral vessels" for the disease that bore his name.

In 1935, Kasanin and Cran reported the first cases of calcifications in the nb visualised on X-rays, an episode that opened up a new path for diagnosis, since calcifications could now be seen in life.

In 1959, Bennet et al. found that in a total of 88 patients with calcifications in the nb, 66% had a history of alterations in phosphorus-calcium metabolism: 42% had primary hypoparathyroidism, 2% post-operative hypoparathyroidism and 16% pseudohypoparathyroidism.On the other hand, in 75 cases of primary hypoparathyroidism, 53% had calcifications in the nb on X-ray. In 31 cases of pseudohypoparathyroidism, 45% also had such calcifications. Clinical analysis of these patients revealed that in 51 patients with altered phosphorus-calcium metabolism (35 with primary hypoparathyroidism, 14 with pseudohypoparathyroidism and 2 in the post-operative period), 70% had convulsions, 63% cataracts, 61% mental retardation and 16% extrapyramidal manifestations, common findings in FD (BENNET et al., 1959).

The studies by Cohen, Duchesnau and Weintein (1980) and Harrington and collaborators (1981), relating intracerebral calcifications to CBCT, confirmed the observations of Bennet and collaborators (1959). CBCT is 15 times more sensitive for diagnosing intracranial calcifications than X-ray, being a casual finding in 0.6% of CT scans (COHEN; DUCHESNAU; WEINTEIN, 1980; HARRINGTON et al., 1981).

In Brazil, the first report of Nb calcifications in the brain dates back to 1981 and described an anatomopathological study of four cases in São Paulo (QUEIROZ;

MALBOUISSON, 1891). Between 1984 and 1986, other cases of BN calcifications were described, but they all had other underlying diseases in common and could not be classified as FD (BRAGA et al., 1985; DELGADO-RODRIGUES, 1984; DIAMENT et al., 1986). The case study by Marilisa Guerreiro and Otoni describes four cases of children with epilepsy and calcifications in the nb. In all the patients described, however, there was no evidence of autosomal dominant disease, but a clinical picture suggestive of pseudohypoparathyroidism, Albright's S. and Hallervorden-Spatz disease (GUERREIRO; OTONI, 1992).

Table 1 shows the articles found in the literature, according to the survey of publications over the last 15 years. The results show that FD has a wide range of clinical findings, with a higher prevalence in females and different genes involved. Table 1 summarises the main findings reported in the selected articles.

Table 1: Literature review on Fahr's disease from 2000 to 2015

ARTICLE	YEAR	COUNTRY	N° OF CASES	AGE	SEX	INITIAL SYMPTOMS	EXAMINATIONS	GENE / LOCALISATION / PROTEIN
Buono et al.	2015	Italy	1	43	F	Chorea, tremor, visual hallucination	CCT - multiple bilateral calcifications in corona radiata, basal nuclei, thalamus and occipital cortex EEG - diffuse delta waves Mini Mental - 22 Biochemistry and haematology - normal	NI
Legati et al.	2015	USA	17	35 a 55 years old	-	Dementia, chorea, ataxia,	CBT - calcifications in the nb, cerebral cortex and cerebellum	XPR1
Nicolas et al.	2014	France	27	Average age 45	-	Mood swings, dementia and ataxia	TCC - calcifications in the dentate nerve, pale gland and striatum	PDGFB
Tuglu et al.	2014	Turkey	1	38	M	Urinary urgency and incontinence, imbalance.	Hormonal and metabolic tests normal, ultrasound, pelvic X-ray and EAS-normal, CCT - calcifications in the nb, in the semioval centre, brainstem, cerebellum and thalamus	NI
Tadke et al.	2014	India	1	25	F	Delirium, dysarthria, cognitive decline	CCT - bilateral calcifications in the nb, oedema in the white and grey matter in the left parietal and occipital regions Liquor - Normal Ca and Mg - normal PTH - low	NI
Hsu et al.	2013	USA	53 members of 29 families	Average age 40	-	Parkinsonism Dystonia Tremor Psychiatric changes	TCC - Bilateral calcifications in the nb, especially in the gl. pallidus Normal metabolic and hormonal exs.	SLC20A2
Nicolas et al.	2013	European Union	32	Average age 45	-	Psychiatric changes, tremor, ataxia	TCC- symmetrical calcifications in the nb	PDGFRB
Wu et al.	2013	USA	1	12	F	Progressive dystonia	Magnetic Resonance Imaging - hypodensity T1	pG521RpT528M

							and T2 in both globes pallidus CBCT - bilateral calcifications in the globes pallidus. Metabolic tests - Normal	
Oliveira and Oliveira	2012	Brazil	3	56	M	Aphasia, atrophy and spasticity	CBT - calcifications in the nb, thalamus, cerebellum and white matter. Normal metabolic and hormonal tests	NI
Shirahama et al.	2010	Japan	3	23	F	Visual hallucination, persecutory delusions, cognitive decline and irritability	TCC - bilateral calcifications in the globus pallidus	NI
Kotan and Aygul	2009	Turkey	6	42	F	Extrapyramidal symptoms and mild metabolic changes	CBT - symmetrical and bilateral calcifications in the NB, thalamus and cerebellum. Normal laboratory tests. Neurological examination - N	NI
Weisman et al.	2007	USA	1	66	M	Slow, progressive cognitive decline at the age of 60 Changes in recent memory, semantic deficits, dysgraphia, aggression	Mini Mental - 30 Laboratory tests - normal CT - diffuse calcifications SPECT - early frontal dementia, hypometabolism in the parietal regions	NI
Modrego et al.	2005	Spain	1	50	F	Progressive dementia	CBCT - calcifications in the nb, cerebellum, semi-oval centre, temporal atrophy MRI - diffuse atrophy greater in the temporal and parietal regions	NI
Pickard et al.	2005	Kingdom United Kingdom and Scotland	2 Mum and daughter		F	Schizophrenia and dementia	TCC - calcifications in the nb FISH - translocation *14q13*	Translocation t (9,14) (q34.2; q13) disruption of the brain transcription factor NPAS3
Cartier et al.	2002	Chile	3	55, 56 e 58	F	Stiffness, ataxia and cognitive impairment from 8, 6 and 10 years old	TCC - Calcifications in the cerebellum, dentate nerve, midbrain, thalamus and semioval centre P3OO - absent Normal laboratory tests	NI
Bobek and Nowak	2000	Poland	2		M	Encephalitis in childhood cognitive impairment, irritability	TCC - extensive calcifications in the nb and cerebellum	NI

Legend: NI - Gene not identified.

In the literature consulted, the nomenclature Idiopathic Base Nucleus *Calcification* or IBGC (*Idiopathic Brain Ganglia Calcification*) was the most commonly used to describe this condition (SOBRIDO et al., 2014). After recent discoveries of the genes involved in 2012, in which mutations were identified, the term FAMILIAL PRIMARY replaced IDIOPATHIC. It is worth noting that the term Fahr's disease is generally used to designate both familial and sporadic calcifications (RAMOS et al., 2004).

Recent studies have identified the genetic basis of FD and made it possible to identify five subtypes: IBGC1, IBGC2, IBGC4 and IBGC5 and IBGC6. The *SLC20A2* gene, located on chromosome 8, contains mutations that cause familial FD. These mutations lead to loss of function of the sodium-dependent phosphate transporter type III (PIT2), which is associated with the disease. The normal protein encoded by this gene (PIT 2) participates in the homeostasis of inorganic phosphate, depending on the coordinated action of parathyroid hormone, vitamin D and fibroblast growth factor 23. The mutations impair phosphate homeostasis and serve as a basis for explaining the molecular aetiology of FD, since the resulting hyperphosphataemia contributes to vascular calcification.

Mutations in the *PDGFRB* and *PDGFB* genes have also been described as causing the disease. These genes are biochemically related: *PDGFBR* codes for the platelet growth factor beta receptor and *PDGFB* codes for the platelet-derived growth factor beta subunit. These genes are active during angiogenesis to recruit pericytes, suggesting that alterations in the blood-brain barrier may be involved in the pathogenesis of this condition (GESCHWIND; LOGINOV; STERN, 1999).

2.2 EPIDEMIOLOGY

It is therefore a rare disease, with an incidence of 1 in 1 million inhabitants, with no defined prevalence, and is more common in women than in men (in a ratio of 2:1). The incidence of basal ganglia calcifications is 0.24 - 2%, with a positive correlation with age (SALEEM et al., 2013).

In patients with FD, symptoms usually start between the ages of 30 and 60, but cases have also been described in children and adolescents. It is important to emphasise that previous studies have shown a suggestive genetic anticipation in affected members of the same family. The age of onset of symptoms decreases by an average of twenty years with each transmission (GESCHWIND; LOGINOV; STERN, 1999).

As an autosomal dominant genetic disease, each child of an affected heterozygous parent has a 50 per cent chance of developing the disease. Combined with the lack of specific treatment and the progressive nature of the disease, the prognosis is poor.

2.3 CLINICAL PRESENTATIONS

A broad clinical spectrum of FD, including extra-pyramidal signs, ataxia, seizures, psychiatric alterations and cognitive decline, has been described in the world and Brazilian literature. One of the factors corroborating this is the large number of articles that are limited to describing isolated cases. Another factor is the heterogeneity in the clinical presentation of genetically proven cases: in the same family there are different clinical manifestations for each individual and even asymptomatic cases (even with positive radiological imaging).

Due to the great variability of clinical signs and symptoms, precise molecular research has become necessary. Mutations in four genes have already been identified as causing FD, namely the *SLC20A2*, *PDGFRB*, *PDGFB and XPR1* genes. Mutations in the *SLC20A2* gene (IBGC1) have been found in more than forty families around the world (HSU et al., 2013; TADIC et al., 2015; WANG et al., 2015) and because it is the most frequent, it will be the focus of genetic research.

2.4 RADIOLOGICAL FINDINGS

There is no clinical-radiological correlation. Members of the same family can have calcifications in the same places with different clinical manifestations or even absence of symptoms.

The most common radiological findings are symmetrical calcifications in the basal nuclei. Rarer tomographic findings include cerebellar calcifications and calcifications in the cortical and subcortical white matter.

The table below summarises the genetic mutations, clinical and radiological findings most commonly found in FD (Table 2):

Table 2: Clinical and radiological findings in the literature according to genetic mutations in FD

CLINICAL FINDINGS	**MUTATION IN *PDGFB* OR *PDGFRB***	***SLC20A2* MUTATION**
CEPHALEA	15 individuals from 2 families	24 individuals from 8 families
ATAXIA	No reports in the literature	20 individuals from 6 families
PSYCHIATRIC DISORDERS	8 individuals from 3 families	28 individuals from 11 families
PARKINSONISM	4 individuals from 3 families	54 individuals from 15 families
KOREA	3 individuals from 1 family	13 individuals from 4 families
RADIOLOGICAL FINDINGS IN TCC	Calcifications in: Basal ganglia, cerebellum, thalamus, cerebral white subst. cerebral white matter, subcortical white matter and dentate nucleus	Calcifications in: Basal ganglia, globus pallidum, thalamus, dentate nucleus, brainstem, cerebral white matter, temporal lobe and cerebellum

Source: OMIM (www.ncbi.nlm.nih.gov)

2.5 GENETIC ASPECTS AND PATHOPHYSIOLOGY

In 1999, the first genetic mapping of a family with basal nucleus calcifications in several generations was carried out. The *locus* was identified on chromosome 14q and the disease was renamed IBGC1 (GESCHWIND; LOGINOV; STERN, 1999). The gene that causes IBGC2 was mapped on chromosome 2q37. IBGC4 is caused by a mutation in the *PDGFRB* gene on chromosome 5q32. IBGC5 is caused by a mutation in the *PDGFB gene on chromosome* 22q12 and IBGC6 is caused by a mutation in the *XPR1* gene on chromosome 1q25. Later, Hsu and colleagues (2013) restudied the first mapped family and identified that the affected individuals had a deleterious mutation in the *SLC20A2* gene and that this mutation was not on chromosome 14, but on chromosome 8, within the *SLC20A2* gene. The term IBGC3 is therefore no longer used.

Genetic advances have revealed that FD is genetically heterogeneous, with six genetic *loci* described. To date, the types described with identified genetic *loci* are those described below in table 3:

Table 3: Types of FD and their genetic *loci*

TYPE I (IBGC1 or PFBC1)	chromosome 8p11.21
TYPE II (IBGC2 or PFBC2)	chromosome 2q37
TYPE IV (IBGC4 or PFBC4)	chromosome 5q32
TYPE V (IBGC5 or PFBC5)	chromosome22q13.3
TYPE VI (IBGC6 or PFBC6)	chromosome1q25

Table 4: Types of Fahr's disease with respective genes involved, chromosomal localisation of genes and proteins encoded

TYPE OF DISEASE	GENE	CHROMOSOMAL LOCUS	PROTEIN
IBGC1	*SLC20A2*	8p11.21	Sodium-dependent phosphate transporter 2
IBGC2	Unknown	2q37	Unknown
IBGC4	*PDGFRB*	5q32	BETA-type receptor for platelet-derived growth factor
IBGC5	*PDGFB*	22q13.1	Subunit B platelet-derived growth factor

Caption: IBGC - *Idiopathic Brain Ganglia Calcification.*

Source: GeneReviews - NCBI Books.

2.6 DIAGNOSTIC CRITERIA

The diagnosis of FD must include all the criteria below, as modified by Moskowitz and Winickoff (1971), Ellie, Julien and Ferrer (1989) and Manyam (2005):

1) Presence of bilateral calcifications in the basal nuclei and/or other brain regions on neuroimaging scans, especially computed tomography of the skull (CT), which easily detects calcium deposits. Other regions can also be affected, such as the cerebellum, semiovale centre and subcortical white matter.

2) Progressive neurological dysfunctions without metabolic, mitochondrial,

biochemical, traumatic, toxic or infectious causes, which generally include movement disorders and/or neuropsychiatric manifestations. Such dysfunctions can be present from childhood, but the most common age of onset is between the fourth and fifth decades of life. Biochemical or metabolic causes should be ruled out after serum tests for calcium, phosphorus, magnesium, alkaline phosphatase, calcitonin and parathormone have been carried out.

(PTH).

3) Family history consistent with autosomal dominant inheritance.

2.7 DIFFERENTIAL DIAGNOSIS

Differential diagnosis should be made mainly with primary and familial forms of autosomal recessive cerebral calcifications, which usually occur with associated endocrine alterations, hypoparathyroidism, pseudo-hypoparathyroidism (caused by mutations in the *GNAS* gene), mitochondrial disorders (MELAS, MERRF, Leigh syndrome), infectious diseases (brucellosis, CM Virus, toxoplasmosis, rubella, cysticercosis), Aicardi- Goutieres syndrome, tuberous sclerosis, Cockayne syndrome, systemic lupus erythematosus and coeliac disease. Table 5 shows the most common aetiologies and causes of cerebral calcifications:

Table 5: Etiologies and most common causes of cerebral calcifications

ETIOLOGY	CAUSE
Genetics	Fahr's disease
Toxic	Carbon monoxide poisoning; lead poisoning
Radio and/or chemotherapy	Secondary mineralising microangiopathy
Infectious	TORCH infections, tuberculosis, AIDS
Metabolic	Hypoparathyroidism Pseudohypoparathyroidism Hyperparathyroidism
Mitochondrial Disease	MELAS, MERRF
Hereditary	Cockayne Syndrome and PKAN

Subtitle: MELAS - *Mitochondrial Encephalomyopathy Lactic Acidosis Stroke-like episodes.* MERRF - *Myoclonic Epilepsy with Ragged Red Fibers.* PKAN - *Pantothenate Kinase Associated Neurodegeneration.* TORCH - Toxoplasmosis, Rubella, Cytomegalovirus and Herpes.

Source: GeneReviews - NCBI Books.

2.6.1 **Differential Diagnosis with Phacomatoses**

Phacomatoses or neuro-ocular-cutaneous syndromes are multi-systemic diseases that include the central nervous system, the eye and skin lesions of varying severity. The presence of cerebral calcifications can occur, but they are usually asymmetrical and associated with cerebral atrophy, data that is not found in FD (RAMOS et al., 2004). Table 6 below shows the location of the calcifications most commonly found in imaging tests for the respective diseases:

Box 6: Calcifications in phacomatoses

Subependymal Nodular Calcification	Tuberous Sclerosis
Calcifications in the Cortical Gyres	Sturge Weber Syndrome
Nodular Calcification in the Cerebellum, Periventricular Regions and Disproportionate Calcification in the Choroid Plexus	Neurofibromatosis
Subependymal Nodular Calcification	Tuberous Sclerosis

2.6.2 **Differential Diagnosis with CNS Infections**

Infections secondary to fungi, bacilli and cestodes can cause meningitis with cerebral calcifications or granulomas. These conditions are usually associated with low immunity and differ from FD by the location of the calcifications or the appearance of a single granuloma (WANG et al., 2015). Table 7 below illustrates the most common diseases and their imaging findings:

Box 7: Calcifications in CNS infections

Calcification in the Leptomeninges	Cryptococcosis or Tuberculosis
Calcified Granuloma in the Brain	Neurocysticercosis, Sarcoid, Tuberculosis

2.6.3 **Differential diagnosis with genetic syndromes**

In FD, the most common laboratory findings are low levels of PTH, vitamin D and serum calcium, constituting hypo- or pseudohypoparathyroidism. Some genetic syndromes have these similarities, but differ in phenotype because they present with malformations, usually in several organs. Another important point is that in these syndromes the calcifications are not as symmetrical as those found in FD (RAMOS et al., 2004). Table 8 below exemplifies some syndromes that present with hypocalcaemia and altered PTH, but have a richer phenotypic picture:

Box 8: Genetic syndromes with resistant hypocalcaemia and PTH alteration

Genetic Sfadromcs that lead to *lesiitcfítc hypoalcsmia* and jlftvjfáo *do ?TH*

Slndromcs	Clinical picture
Hereditary Aibright Osteodystrophy (Pspu cÈohi po parati reoi riisma)	DM, short stature, epilepsy, basal ganglia ealdrophy, PTHf
Di George's sequel	Thymus, thyroid, parathyroid and great vessels defects

(H ipo for tircoidi smo+M eiífor iraç õcs)	
Linear Arrow Nevus Sequence	Hyperkeratosis fadai epilepsy, vitamin 0-resistant menchitis
Sindrpme d? Shprintzen	DM, short stature, heart defect, cleft palate
Congenital hypoparathyroidism	1 Isolaria = hspacalcmia, PTH 2- Familial = recessive or dominant requires family history 3- Autoimmune = associated with endocirrhotic diseases

□M, Llí-fn.iíiRiA íriPTítA:, HH, hofíMmfl param

Source: MedicinaNET (http://www.medicinanet.com.br/conteudos/revisoes/5616/hiperparatireoidismo)

CHAPTER 3

OBJECTIVES

Analysing a rare disease, Fahr's disease, by means of a case study, including research into its relatives (the father and his sisters).

Carry out a genetic study of this family in order to identify the gene involved, focusing on *SLC20A2, a* gene commonly related to the disease.

CHAPTER 4

MATERIAL AND METHODS

4.1 MATERIAL

The proband, her father and her younger sisters were included in this neuroclinical study. The proband's clinical data was obtained from her medical records and through laboratory tests carried out by the Unified Health System. The radiological assessment included skull CT scans of the aforementioned limbs and MRI scans of the proband's brain, which were carried out respectively at the Alcides Carneiro School Hospital and the Santa Tereza Hospital in Petrópolis, under agreement with the SUS. The genetic tests included karyotyping, FISH, a-CGH and were carried out only on the proband. These tests were carried out by geneticist Dr Cassio Luiz Carvalho Serrão (Alcides Carneiro Hospital, Petrópolis, RJ).

4.2 ETHICAL ASPECTS

The patient's carer signed the Informed Consent Form (ICF) (APPENDIX A), agreeing to take part in the study. Based on this data, the family heredogram was created using a specific programme (GenoPro - www.genopro.com).

The study was approved by the Research Ethics Committee of the Federal University of Rio de Janeiro (UNIRIO) under CAAE number: 74660717.0.0000.5258.

4.3 ANALYSING MEDICAL RECORDS, CLINICAL AND LABORATORY TESTS

The author analysed the medical records and collected data from the anamnesis and complementary tests carried out by the proband since the onset of symptoms. Her parents and younger sisters took part in the interviews in person and by telephone, and blood tests (blood count, electrolytes, thyroid hormone and PTH assessment, EAS, glycaemia, lipidogram) were carried out at the Alcides Carneiro Hospital laboratory. The physical examination included inspection, assessment of dynamic balance and a full neurological examination. The EEG was carried out on the proband, her sisters and her father, also by SUS. Imaging tests (CBCT and MRI) were restricted to symptomatic patients.

The preliminary genetic tests were karyotyping, sequencing of the *SLC20A2* gene to search for variants of this gene (by extracting DNA from peripheral blood cells followed by DNA analysis using NEXT GENERATION SEQUENCING - NGS, using the illumina platform), FISH (using a specific probe for chromosome 8, with analysis of 200 nuclei in fluorescence equipment) and chromosome analysis by MICROARRAY (extraction of DNA from peripheral blood, followed by cytogenomic analysis by comparative hybridisation of proband DNA marked with the Cy5 fluorophore versus control DNA marked with the Cy3 fluorophore with 180,000 probes arranged on a Microarray platform). The tests were carried out by the DLE laboratory in Rio de Janeiro, with the exception of FISH, which was carried out by the Álvaro laboratory (Petrópolis - RJ).

Figure 1 below exemplifies the CGH-Array process.

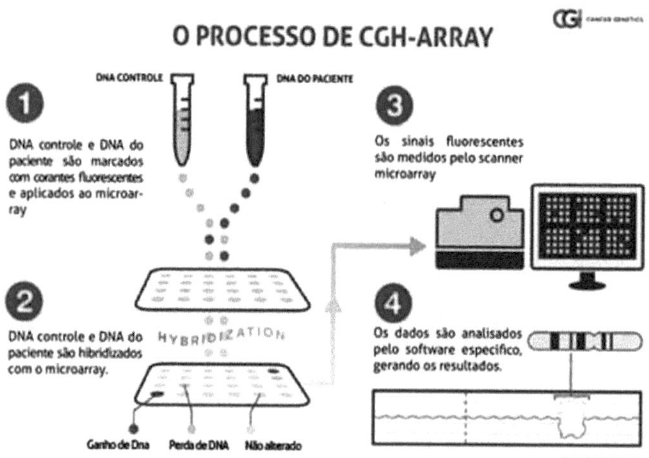

Figure 1: CGH-Array test. Item 4 exemplifies a deletion
Source: Hermes Pardini Laboratory

CHAPTER 5

RESULTS

A 10-year-old white girl from Rio de Janeiro, the eldest child of a non-consanguineous couple, attending primary school, was taken by her mother for the first time to the neurology outpatient clinic because she presented frequent seizures of the Absence type, a decline in school performance and intense headaches, accompanied by phonation and photophobia. The neurological examination at the time showed no alterations, but the EEG revealed excessive delta activity in the temporal regions (rs), with a predominance on the right. Diagnosed as epileptic, she was treated with oxcarbazepine and valproic acid and remained seizure-free for two years.

Of note, in his previous history he had had two episodes of convulsive seizures with fever; at 8 months and 2 years and 4 months, both generalised atonic seizures. The electroencephalogram and skull X-ray at the time were normal. At the time, the medication chosen was phenobarbital drops, but the proband developed a skin allergy and the treatment was suspended. The anamnesis also revealed that she had been born in a dystocia, and had developed a slight motor delay. Initial neurological and physical examinations showed no alterations.

At the age of 12, the mother returned with the proband, who was scattered, with slight gait ataxia and reported dizziness. The EEG revealed no alterations. The following year, her school performance worsened, as did her headaches, which were temporally localised and refractory to common analgesics. Due to the absence of seizures, the medication was changed to topiramate. The clinical picture continued for two years, with no objective improvement. At the end of 2014, he returned to the clinic complaining of dizziness, worsening headaches and hand tremors. A new neurological examination showed mild muscle hypotonia, fine motor incoordination, bilateral hand tremor, which worsened with force manoeuvres, Chvostek's sign (Figure 2), ataxic gait, mild dysmetria and slow comprehension. In view of the clinical worsening and the cerebellar condition, a more accurate diagnostic investigation was necessary. Nuclear magnetic resonance imaging of the brain was then requested, which showed punctate calcifications in the thalamus, dentate nuclei in the white matter of the frontal and parietal lobes and in the cerebellum (Figure 3). Given this information, the mother informed us that the father had a CT scan of the skull with similar characteristics and was taking anticonvulsants. This information raised the hypothesis of a genetic disease

The family was referred to the genetics department at the Alcides Carneiro Hospital. New laboratory and electrographic tests were also requested for the proband, as shown in Table 9 below and Figures 4 and 5:

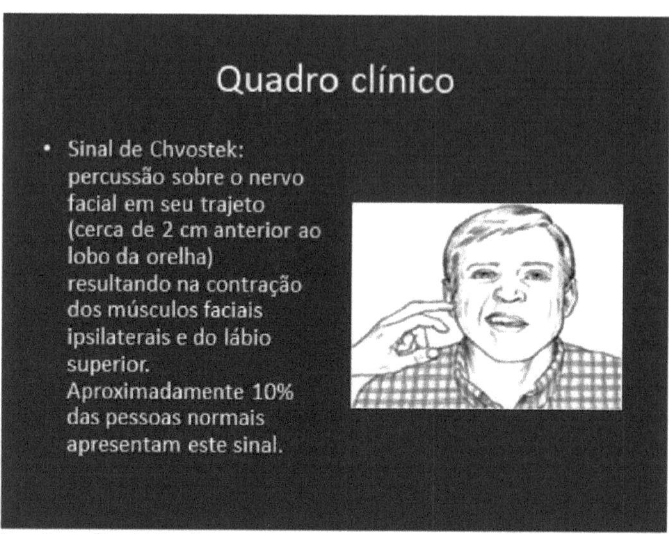

Figura 2: Chvostek Signal

Source: MedicinaNET (medicinanet.com.br/conteudos/revisoes/5617/hipoparathyroidism.htm)

Table 9: Summary of laboratory and EEG findings

Tests	Date of realisation	Standard Result	Result Found
EEG	12/2011	normal	Temporal delta wave paroxysms
	6/2012 e 11/2013		Normal
	3/2015		Bilateral F-T-C theta waves
	3/2016		Bilateral F-C theta waves
Total Calcium	5/2015		6.3mg /dl
	7/2015	8.8 to 11mg/dl	10.4mg/dl
	12/2015		8.6 mg/dl
	4/2016		8.5mg/dl
24-hour urinary calcium	5/2015	Less than 250 mg/24 hrs	0.3 and 7.2mg /24hrs
	12/2015		30 mg/ 24 hrs
Vit D 25 hydroxy	5/2015		35.20 mg/ml
	7/2015	30-100mg/ml	25.2 mg/ml
	12/2015		38.5 mg/ml
	4/2016		30.05mg/ml
Phosphorus	5/2015		7.8 mg/dl
	7/2015	2.54.8 mg/dl	5.9 mg/dl
	12/2015		5.3 mg/dl
	4/2016		5.6mg/dl
Serum magnesium	5/2015		1.83mg/dl
	7/2015	1.58-2.56 mg/dl	2.04mg/dl
	12/2015		1.97mg/dl
Parathormone	4/2016		1.98mg/dl
	5/2015	15-65 picograms per millilitre	6.00pg/ml
	7/2015		7.5 pg/ml
	12/2015		13pg/ml

	4/2016		13.5pg/ml
Thyroid Exs (T3, T4, TSH)	5/2015	70-205 ng/dl	normal
	7/2015	4.5-12.8 ug/dl	normal
	12/2015	Up to 4.9ng/dl	normal
	4/2016		normal

Source: SUS

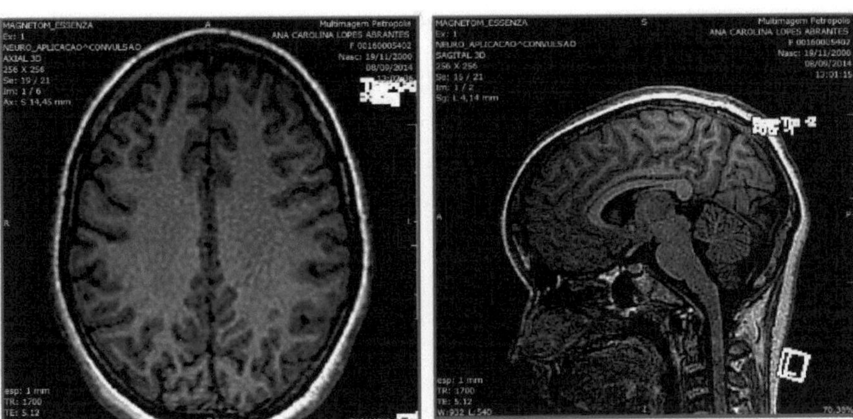

Figura 3: Magnetic resonance imaging of the proband's brain - September 2014

Source: Santa Teresa Hospital Imaging Service - SUS

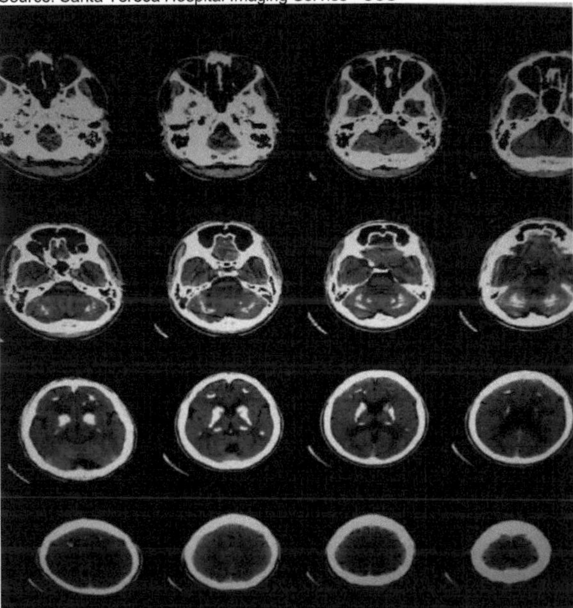

Figura 4: Magnetic resonance imaging of the proband's brain - October 2016

Source: Santa Teresa Hospital Imaging Service - SUS

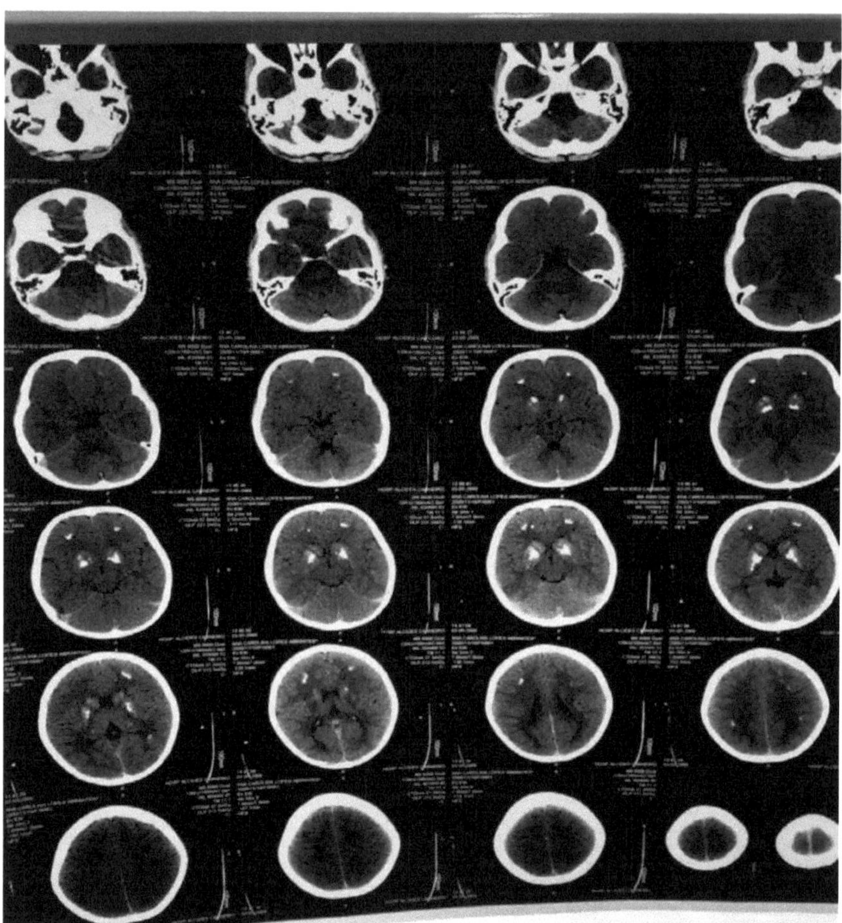

Figure 5: CT scan of the proband's skull - July 2016

Source: Alcides Carneiro Hospital Imaging Service - SUS

The geneticist's anamnesis revealed that the patient's father had been suffering from seizures since he was five years old and had been treated with phenobarbital. In adolescence, he developed fine motor incoordination and dizziness, and later had manual tremor that worsened with forceful manoeuvres. On examination, he also had corneal opacification and convergent strabismus in his right eye. A brain MRI carried out in March 2015 showed alterations characteristic of Fahr's disease: symmetrical calcifications in the basal nuclei and cerebellar lobes, gliosis in the caudate nucleus, corona radiata, periventricular white matter and deep white matter of the right frontal lobe, signs of accentuation of basal cisterns, cisuras and convexity grooves, with proportional ectasia of the ventricular system. The EEG showed slow waves in the theta range, excessive and diffuse, with greater expression in the bilateral temporal regions. Despite being medicated, he still had atonic seizures. The anamnesis also revealed that two of the proband's paternal uncles had seizures, without having carried out any more in-depth investigations. The couple's second and third daughters were initially healthy, asymptomatic and had normal laboratory tests. There was no relevant data in the mother's history.

Figure 6 shows the family's heredogram and Table 10 summarises the clinical findings of hypoparathyroidism. Neuromuscular and ocular alterations were found in the physical examination of the father.

HEREDOGRAMA

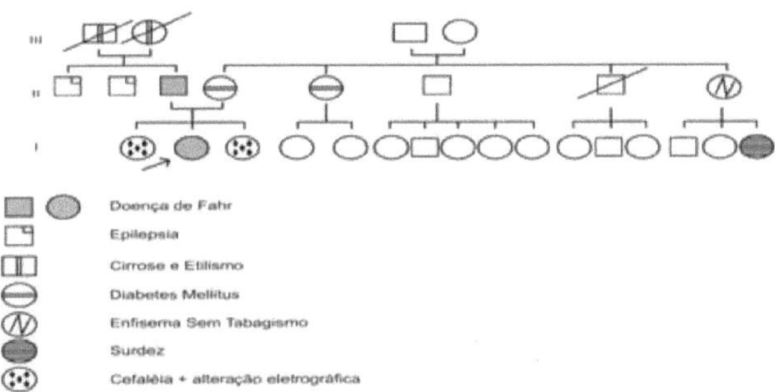

Figure 6: Heredogram of the proband

Source: Heredogram produced online at http://www.genopro.com/ for genealogies (GenoPro)

Box 10: Clinical findings of hypoparathyroidism

Neuromuscular: cramps, tetany, myalgia (including chest pain), muscle weakness, paresthesia (in the fingers and perioral area), carpopedal spasm, Trousseau's and Chvostek's signs.

Skin and glands: dry skin, hair loss, alopecia

Neurological: parkinsonism, dysarthria, gait alterations, postural instability, convulsions

Ocular: pseudopapitedema, cataract

Cardiovascular: ST segment and QT interval prolongation, electrocardiogram changes suggestive of acute myocardial infarction, arrhythmias, heart failure

Dental: enamel hypoplasia, dentin defects, delayed tooth eruption, cavities, shortened molar roots and eventually loss of all teeth

Respiratory: laryngospasm, bronchospasm

Source: MedicinaNET (http://www.medicinanet.com.br/conteudos/revisoes/5616/hiperparatireoidismo)

Given the data from the anamnesis and family history, and the alterations in the physical and radiological examinations of the proband and her genitor that pointed to an autosomal dominant disease, more specific genetic tests were carried out on the proband:

- G-band karyotype: 46, XX;
- Sequencing of the *SLC20A2* GENE, chromosomal location 8p11.21 - NO point mutations or small insertions or deletions with known clinical relevance were detected in the coding region of the *SLC20A2 gene;*
- FISH (*Fluorescent In Situ Hybridisation*) - reciprocal chromosomal translocation of the long arms of chromosomes 9 and 22-t (9;22) was detected. It should be noted that the patient had no clinical and/or laboratory signs of chronic leukaemia.
- Array-CGH (a-CGH) test: no copy number variations were observed on chromosomes 9 and 22.

As the study progressed, the patient's condition worsened with depression and headache. The EEG performed in August 2017 showed excessive theta waves in the bilateral temporo-central regions, without worsening seizures. She was medicated with Oxcarbazepine 600 mg/day and Sodium Divalproate 600 mg/day. The CBT from the same period (Figure 7) revealed coarse calcifications in the nb, putamen, pale gls, thalamus and subcortical regions of the frontal and parietal lobes, and punctate calcifications in the cerebellar dentate nuclei. Her two sisters began to suffer from chronic headaches. The CCTs of both were normal, but the EEGs showed alterations of an epileptogenic nature (Figure 8), with no signs of seizures. The father evolved with significant cognitive decline and psychiatric alterations such as heteroaggression and hypersexuality.

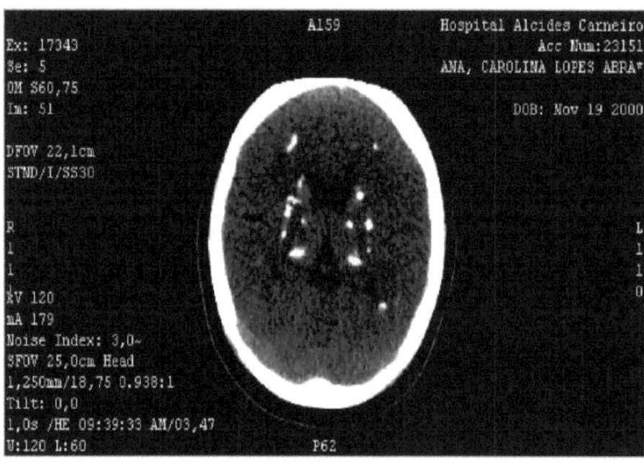

Figure 7: proband's Capstone - August 2017

Source: Alcides Carneiro Hospital Imaging Service - SUS

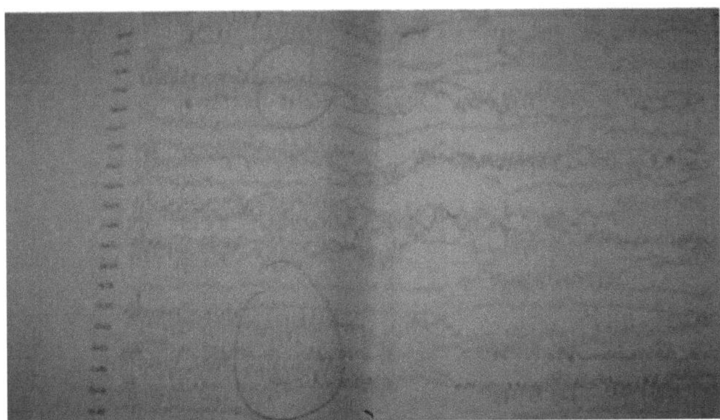

Figure 8: EEG of the proband's older sister - August 2017

CHAPTER 6

DISCUSSION

This dissertation describes an extremely rare case of an adolescent with an initial diagnosis of epilepsy who evolved with cerebellar signs, worsening seizures and cognitive decline, whose neuroimaging and laboratory tests, together with a positive family history for autosomal dominant disease, were consistent with FD.

Our literature review found 16 articles describing 25 cases, 19 of which belonged to the same group of families (Chart 1). Similar to this dissertation, all the articles were case reports. It is important to highlight the work by Hsu et al. (2013) which showed the study of 29 families with FD and evidence that 9 of the 14 mutations identified in the *SLC20A2* gene introduced a stop codon, pointing to haploinsufficiency as a causal mechanism for familial FD (HSU et al., 2013). All the patients included had cerebral calcifications in the basal nuclei, cerebral cortex, cerebellum and thalamus, with a higher incidence in the globus pallidus. Only two cases had isolated calcifications in the basal nuclei.

CBCT was the test that best identified the imaging findings in our proband and in the cases reviewed in the literature. Also in this context, laboratory tests pointed to hypocalcaemia with low PTH levels, configuring hypoparathyroidism (also seen in our report, see table 9). There was a prevalence of females (eighteen women to seven men) and an average age of occurrence between the fourth and fifth decades. The most frequent signs and symptoms were extrapyramidal and dementia, followed by psychiatric alterations. The rarest symptoms described were headache (BUONO et al., 2015; TADKE et al. 2014) urinary incontinence (TUGLU et al., 2014) and convulsion (BUONO et al., 2015). There was equivalence between the clinical and laboratory phenotypes. Penetrance, on the other hand, proved to be incomplete and age-related: in the case of anatomical alteration, there was 95% penetrance in patients aged 50 or over, and in the case of clinical alteration, no more than 70% penetrance. Molecular genetic evaluation through sequencing of the identified gene and FISH and a-CGH tests revealed *locus* heterogeneity: a description of mutations in the enzyme encoded by the paternal and maternal hereditary neurodegeneration genes (respectively *PG521R* and *PT528M*) (WU et al., 2013) and a case of positive FISH for 14q13 involving the NPAS3 transcription factor (PICKARD et al., 2005). The *SLC20A2* gene was identified in 2012 and located on chromosome 8, which contains a mutation causing familial Fahr's disease. This mutation leads to a loss of function of the "*type III sodium dependent phosphate transporter 2* (PIT2) which is associated with the disease. The genetic evaluation of our patient showed no alterations in the *SLC20A2* gene and no variations in chromosomes 9 and 22.

In patients with FD, calcium deposits can be found in the putamen and caudate nuclei, internal capsule, globus pallidus, dentate nucleus, thalamus, cerebellum and cerebral white matter. Histopathological analysis usually reveals concentric calcium deposits in the basal nuclei, white matter, cerebellum, inside the walls of small and medium calibre arteries and, less frequently, in veins. The calcifications found in the father's CCT were located in the nb and cerebellum, associated with gliosis in the white matter of the right frontal lobe, the caudate nucleus and the corona radiata. Signs of cortical atrophy were present. The proband's last CCT revealed radiological worsening, consistent with the clinical worsening: coarse calcifications in the nb, putamen, pale gls, thalamus, subcortical rs of the frontal and parietal lobes, as well as punctate calcifications in the cerebellar dentate nb.

FD can also be asymptomatic. This fact is important because it shows that the brain circuits may have intact function despite the parenchymal deposition of substances, indicating the possible existence of other causal factors for the alterations described (KUMMER et al., 2006).

It is important to point out that the literature on FD is problematic because it includes, under the name of Fahr's syndrome, other conditions that have pathological calcification, i.e. not idiopathic, in the basal nuclei (KUMMER et al., 2006).

Idiopathic hypoparathyroidism is characterised by hypocalcaemia with low or non-existent PTH levels. The early form can occur due to failure in the development of the parathyroid gland, due to congenital agenesis or hypoplasia, causing neonatal hypoparathyroidism. In these cases, hypoparathyroidism can be isolated (autosomal recessive or X-linked) or associated with thymus aplasia and cardiac anomalies (Di George Syndrome). In the proband's case, there was no history of neonatal hypoparathyroidism or other associated anomalies, justifying ruling out these diagnostic hypotheses. In autoimmune polyglandular syndromes, other hormonal alterations are present (TSH, GH, prolactin), which were not found in the proband (GOUVEIA et al., 2010). In activating mutations of the calcium-sensing receptor gene, hypercalciuria is present, which was also not found in the proband's tests. In all these cases, the phenotypic alterations are more evident and do not present with cerebral calcifications, which is fundamental for the hypothesis of FD. PTH resistance syndromes (Pseudohypoparathyroidism type I or Albright Osteodystrophy and type II) are also causes of hypocalcaemia and cerebral calcifications, but with increased PTH levels due to the target organs being unresponsive to its biological action. In this group of diseases, bone abnormalities, short stature, syndromic fasciitis and mental deficiency are present, data that was not found in the proband.

There are many diseases that occur with cerebral calcifications, as mentioned above. However, the positive family history of the father, who presented with progressive seizures, cognitive decline, cerebellar signs and subsequent confirmation with imaging tests left no doubt as to the autosomal dominant nature with incomplete penetrance and variable expressiveness of the disease.

During the five years of follow-up in the neurology clinic, the progressive and worsening nature of the disease became clear. The proband, who initially had sparse seizures that were easily controlled with monotherapy, progressed with worsening seizures, cognitive decline and cerebellar signs (dizziness, gait ataxia and manual tremor). The initial hypothesis of epilepsy then merited more thorough radiological and laboratory investigation. The results of the tests, together with the family history, led to the diagnostic conclusion.

Due to the wide range of signs and symptoms that FD has and the large number of other diseases that occur with hypoparathyroidism, precise molecular research is mandatory. Despite the difficulties in obtaining these tests through the Unified Health System (SUS), the persistence of the mother and the diagnostic importance corroborated the consent of the courts, through the Public Defender's Office, to carry them out. Unfortunately, so far it has not been possible to carry out a genetic evaluation of the father, who is the probable carrier of the mutation that causes the disease.

Also considering the literature survey, it was found that mutations in the *SLC20A2* gene were the most commonly found worldwide (WANG et al., 2015), which is why our first genetic focus was on this gene. Contradictorily, the sequencing of this gene carried out on the proband was negative, as were the FISH and a-CGH tests, which also showed no molecular alterations. In the future, we will try to carry out exome sequencing, a method that evaluates 80% of all exons (coding regions), in order to investigate mutations in other genes to complete the molecular diagnosis and then carry out accurate genetic counselling.

7 CONCLUSIONS

The patient in this study has a clinical picture, evolution, laboratory tests and imaging compatible with FD, and is, as far as we know, the first case described in the city of Rio de Janeiro.

Brain calcifications can occur in physiological conditions and in other diseases, with or without neuropsychiatric symptoms and signs. CBT status may not fully reflect the state of the disease. This can be explained by the fact that non-specific calcifications are often present in older individuals and are generally absent in younger members of the affected family (KUMMER et al., 2006). However, when such findings occur symmetrically and in more than one family member, coexisting with a wide range of symptoms and signs, it is important to consider FD as a potential diagnosis.

Although there is no cure for FD, the likelihood of 50% of descendants being affected and the progressive nature of the disease reinforce the need for an accurate diagnosis for subsequent genetic counselling. The clinical and laboratory findings found in FD are not pathognomonic of the disease. Cerebral calcifications in nb are more symmetrical and numerous than those found in the other alterations described in the differential diagnosis, but they are not exclusive to FD. These points justify the need for molecular genetic research and show the relevance of this study.

The genetic evaluation of our patient showed no alterations in the *SLC20A2* gene or variations in chromosomes 9 and 22.

FINAL CONSIDERATIONS

The proband and her family continue to be monitored at the neurology clinic. She and her genitor will have to undergo further molecular research into other genes and/or exome sequencing to identify the mutation that causes FD.

REFERENCES

BAMBERGER, H. Beobachtungen und bemerkungen uber hirnkrankheiten. *Verhandl Phy Med Ges.*, [S.l.], v. 6, p. 325-8, 1855.

BENNET, J.C.; MAFFLY, R.H.; STEINBACH, H.L.The Significance of Bilateral Basal Ganglia Calcification. *Radiology*, [S.l.], v. 72, p. 368-378, 1959.

BOBEK, J.; NOWAK, M. Familial Form of Fahr Syndrome (Report of two Cases). *Neurological Neurochir Pol*, [S.l.], v. 34, n. 1, p. 167-75, 2000.

BRAGA, F.M.; ZUKERMAN, E.; FERRAZ, I.A.P.; VIRTTUZZO, R. Intense and Symmetrical Calcifications of the Basal Ganglia and Cerebellum Visualised on Computed Tomography of the Skull. *Arq Bras Neurocirurgia*, [S.l.], v. 4, p. 115-122, 1985.

BUONO, V.; CORALLO, F.; COSTA, A.; BRAMANTI, P.; MARINO, S. Quantitative MR Markers and Psychiatric Symptoms in a Patient with Fahr Disease. *Am J Case Rep*, [S.l.], v. 16, p. 382-5, 2015.

CARTIER, L.; PASSIG, C.; GORMAZ, A.; LÓPEZ, J. Nueropsychological and Neurophysiological Features of Fahr's Disease. *Rev Med Chile*, [S.l.], v. 130, n. 12, p. 1383-90, 2002.

COHEN, C.R.; DUCHESNAU, P.M.; WEINTEIN, M.A. Calcification of the Basal Ganglia as visualised by Tomography. *Radiology*, [S.l.], v. 134, p. 97-99, 1980.

DELACOUR, A . Ossification of the capillaires du cerveau. *Ann Med Psychol.*, [S.l.], v. 2, p. 458-61, 1850.

DELGADO-RODRIGUES, R.N. Neurocysticercosis associated with hypoparathyroidism and Fahr's disease: report of a case. *Arq Neuropsiquiatr.*, São Paulo, v. 42, p. 388391, 1984.

DIAMENT, A.J.; MACHADO, L.R.; CYPEL, S.; RAMOS, J.L.A. Syndrome of basal ganglia calcification, leukodystrophy and chronic lymphomonocytic pleiocytosis in cerebrospinal fluid. *Arq Neuropsiquiatr.*, São Paulo, v. 44, p. 185190, 1986.

ELLIE, E.; JULIEN, J.; FERRER, X. Familial idopathic striopallioentate calcifications. *Neurology*, [S.l.], v. 39, p. 381-85, 1989.

FAHR, T. Idiopathische Verkalkung der Hirngefã^e. *Zentralbl Allg Pathol.,* [S.l.], v. 50, p. 129-33, 1930.

GESCHWIND, D.H.; LOGINOV, M.; STERN, J.M. Identification of a Locus on Chromosome 14 q for Idiopathic Basal Ganglia Calcification (Fahr Disease). *Am J Hum Genet*, [S.l.], v. 65, p. 764-72, 1999.

GOUVEIA, S.; RIBEIRO, C.; GOMES, L.; CARVALHEIRO, M. Autoimmune polyglandular syndrome type 2; clinical-laboratory characterisation and recommendations for approach and follow-up. *Revista Portuguesa de Endocrinologia*, [S.l.], p. 69-82, 2010.

GUERREIRO, M.M.; OTONI, A.E. Calcifications of the Basal Ganglia in Childhood. *Arq Neuropsiquiatr.*, [S.l.], v. 50, p. 513-518, 1992.

HSU, S.C.; SEARS, R.L.; LEMOS, R.R.; QUITANS, B.; HUANG, A.; SPITERI, E.; et al. Mutations in SLC20A2 are a Major Cause of Familial Idiopathic Basal Ganglia Calcification. *Neurogenetics*, [S.l.], v. 14, p. 11-22, 2013.

KASANIN, J.; CRAN, K.R.P. A Case of Extensive Calcification of the Brain: selective calcification of the finer cerebral blood vessels. *Arch Neurol.*, [S.l.], v. 34, p. 164-178, 1962.

KOTAN, D.; AYGUL, R. Familial Fahr Disease in a Turkish Family. *South Medical Journal*, [S.l.], v. 102, n. 1, p. 85-6, 2009.

KUMMER, A.; DE CASTRO, M.; CARAMELLI, P.; CARDOSO, F.; TEIXEIRA, A.L. Severe behavioural changes in patients with Fahr's disease. *Arq Neuropsiquiatr.*, [S.l.], v. 64, n. 3-A, p. 645-649, 2006.

LEGATI, A.; GIOVANNINI, D.; NICOLAS, G.; et al. Mutation in XPR1 causes Primary Familial Brain Calcification associated with altered phosphate export. *Nat Genetic*, [S.l.], v. 47, n. 6, p. 579-581, 2015.

MANYAM, B.V. What is and what is not Fahr's Disease. *Parkinsonism Relat Disord*, [S.l.], v. 11, p. 73-80, 2005.

MODREGO, P.J.; MOJONERO, J.; SERRANO, M.; FAYED, N. Fahr's Syndrome Presenting With Pure and Progressive Presenile Dementia. *Neurol Sci* , [S.l.], v. 26, n. 5, p. 637-9, 2005.

MOSKOWITZ, M.A.; WINICKOFF, H.E.R. Familial Calcification of the Basal Ganglia: a metabolic and genetic study. *N Engl J Med*, [S.l.], v. 285, p. 72-7, 1971.

NICOLAS, G.; JACQUIN, A.; THAUVIN-ROBINET, C.; et al. A de novo nonsense PDGFB mutation causing Idiopathic Basal Ganglia Calcification with Laryngeal Dystonia. *Eur J Hum Genet*, [S.l.], v. 22, p. 1236-1238, 2014.

NICOLAS, G.; POTTIER, C.; COUTANT, S.; et al. Mutation of the PDGFRB gene as a cause of Idiopathic Basal Ganglia Calcification. *Neurology*, [S.l.], v. 80, p. 181-187, 2013.

OLIVEIRA, M.F.; OLIVEIRA, J.R.M. A Comorbid Case of Familial Idiopathic Basal Ganglia Calcification (Fahr Disease) Associated With Post-Polio Syndrome. *The Journal of Neuropsychiatry,* [S.l.], v. 24, n. 2, p. 14-15, 2012.

PICKARD, B.S.; MALLOY, M.P.; PORTEOUS,D.J.; BLACKWOOD, D.H.; MUIR, W.J. American Journal of Med Genetic B. *Neuropsychiatric Genet*, [S.l.], v. 136B, n.1, p. 26-32, 2005.

QUEIROZ, A.C.; MALBOUISSON, A.M.B. Calcification of the Basal Nuclei in the Brain: an anatomopathological study of 4 cases. *Arq Neuropsiquiatr.*, São Paulo, v. 39, p. 321-326, 1981.

SALEEM, S.; ASLAM, H.M.; ANWAR, M.; ANWAR, S.; SALEE, M.; SALEEM, A.; REHMANI, M.A.K. Farh's Syndrome: Literature Review of Current Evidence. *Orphanet J Rare Disease*, [S.l.], v. 8, p. 156, 2013.

SHIRAHAMA, M.; AKIYOSHI, J.; ISHITOBI, Y.; TANAKA, Y.; TSURU, J.; MATSUSHITA, H.; HANADA, H.; KODAMA, K. A Young Woman With Visual Hallucination Delusions of

Persecution and a History of Performing Arson with Possible Three-Generation Fahr Disease. *Acta Psychiatric Scand*, [S.l.], v. 121, n. 1, p. 75-7, 2010.

SOBRIDO, M.J.; COPPOLA, G.; OLIVEIRA, J.; HOPFER, S; GESCHWIND, D.H. *Primary Familial Brain Calcification*. Gene Reviews, 2014.

RAMOS, E.M.; OLIVEIRA, J.; SOBRIDO, M.J.; COPPOLA, G. *Primary Familial Brain Calcification*. In: ADAM, M.P.; ARDINGER, H.H.; PAGON, R.A.; et al. GeneReviews, Seattle (WA): University of Washington, 2004.

TADIC, V.; WESTENBERGER, A.; DOMINGO, A.; ALVAREZ-FISHER, D.; KLEIN, C.; KASTEN, M. Primary Brain Calcification With Known Gene Mutations. A Systematic Review and Challenges of Phenotypic Characterisation. *JAMA Neurol*, [S.l.], v. 72, n. 4, p. 460-7, 2015.

TADKE, R.; FAYE, A.D.; GAWANDE, S.; KIRPEKAR, V.C.; BHAVE, S.H. A Case Report of Psychosis due to Fahr's Syndrome and Response to Behavioural Disturbances with Risperidone and Oxcarbazepine. *Indian J Psychiatry*, [S.l.], v. 56., n. 2, p. 188-90, 2014.

TUGLU, D.; YUVANÇ, E.; BAL, F.; TURKEL, Y.; DAG, E.; YILMAZ, E.; BATISLAM, E. Fahr Syndrome Unknown Complication: Overactive Bladder. *Case Rep Urol.*, [S.l.], p. 939268, 2014.

WANG, H.; SHAO, B.; WANG, L.; YE, Q. Fahr's disease in two siblings in a family: A case report. *Exp Ther Med.*, [S.l.], v. 9, n. 5, p. 1931-3, 2015.

WEISMAN, D.C.; YAARI, R.; HANSEN, L.A.; THAL, L.J. Density of the brain, decline of the mind: an atypical case of Fahr disease. *Arch of Neurology*, v. 64, n. 5, p. 7567, 2007.

WU, Y.W.; HESS, C.P.; SINGHAL, N.S.; GRODEN,C.; TORO, C. Idiopathic basal ganglia calcifications: an atypical presentation of PKAN. *Pediatric Neurology*, [S.l.], v. 49, n. 5, p. 351-4, 2013.

APPENDIX A - Informed Consent Form

INFORMED CONSENT FORM

You are being invited as a volunteer to take part in the research: please enter the title of the survey.
CASE REPORT OF AN ADOLESCENT WITH FAHR DISEASE under the supervision of master's student **DRA. CRISTIANE MARINS FERREIRA** and under the responsibility of researcher **Profª . CARMEN LÚCIA ANTÃO PAIVA, from UNIRIO - FEDERAL UNIVERSITY OF THE STATE OF RIO DE JANEIRO,** Department of Postgraduate Neurology.

BACKGROUND, OBJECTIVES AND PROCEDURES: The reason for studying this case is to analyse the clinical and radiological aspects of Fahr's disease. The research is justified because it is a rare disease, with few cases described in the Brazilian literature. It is also relevant because it is an accurate neurogenetic assessment carried out in the Unified Health System, which can guide studies for future treatment. The aim of this project is to identify the affected gene for subsequent genetic counselling of the family.
The procedure(s) for collecting material will be as follows: peripheral blood will be collected from the proband and their family members by the neurologist and geneticists, in their own hospital environment, at no cost to the participants. Data and interviews will be carried out by Dr Cristiane Marins by telephone or direct anamnesis on a weekly basis.

DISCOURTS, RISKS AND BENEFITS: there is minimal discomfort and risk for you who will be subjected to the collection of material (drawing of blood) for the laboratory and genetic tests, which is justified by the benefit that the results will bring for an accurate diagnosis.

FORM OF MONITORING AND ASSISTANCE: the patient and her immediate family will be monitored by Dr Cassio Luiz Serão and Dr Cristiane Marins. Any clinical complications that may occur during the study will also be dealt with by the aforementioned doctors. Any questions you or your family members may have should be clarified with Dr Cristiane Marins (tel. 24992955923).

GUARANTEE OF DISCLOSURE, FREEDOM OF REFUSAL AND GUARANTEE OF SECILITY: you will be informed about the research in any way you wish. You are free to refuse to participate, withdraw your consent or stop participating at any time. Your participation is voluntary and refusal to participate will not result in any penalty or loss of benefits.
Your identity will be treated with professional standards of confidentiality. The results of all the tests carried out and the study will be sent to you if you wish. Your name or material indicating your participation will not be released without your permission. You will not be identified in any publication that may result from this study. A copy of this informed consent will be filed with the Neurology Postgraduate Programme at the Federal University of Rio de Janeiro and another will be provided to you. RCTs and information/data

obtained from the research will be stored safely for five years and then disposed of in an environmentally friendly way.

PARTICIPATION COSTS, REIMBURSEMENT AND INDEMNIFICATION FOR ANY DAMAGES: Participation in the study will not entail any costs for you and no additional financial compensation will be made available beyond that provided for in the project budget.

DECLARATION BY THE PARTICIPANT OR THE PERSON RESPONSIBLE FOR THE PARTICIPANT:
I, CONCEIÇÃO LOPES LEITE, parent and guardian of participant ANA CAROLINA LOPES ABRANTES, have been informed of the objectives of the above research in a clear and detailed manner and have clarified my doubts. I know that at any time I can request new information and **change** my decision if I so wish. **The student**, the supervising professor CARMEN LÚCIA ANTÃO PAIVA and the co-supervising professor DRA. REGINA MARIA PAPAIS ALVARENGA have assured me that all personal details will remain confidential.
If you have any questions, you can call Dr Cristiane Marins Ferreira on (24) 992955923 **or the HUGG Ethics Committee (21 2264-5177), Rua Mariz e Barros, 775, Tijuca. Rio de Janeiro. CEP 20.270-004. Entrance via Orthopaedics, 4th floor)**. I declare that I agree to my daughter taking part in this study. I have received a copy of this informed consent form and have been given the opportunity to read it and clarify my doubts.

ANA CAROLINA LOPES ABRANTES/ CONCEIÇÃO LOPES LEITE

.... //.......
Participant's name Signature Date

CARMEN LÚCIA ANTÃO PAIVA.

.... //.......
Researcher's name Signature Date
Phone: (21 22645177) HUGG - Rua Mariz e Barros, 775. Tijuca. Rio de Janeiro. CEP 20.270-004. Entrance via Orthopaedics, 4th floor).

CRISTIANE MARINS FERREIRA

.... //.......
Name of student-researcher Signature Date
Phone: (24) 994476046
HUGG-Rua Mariz e Barros, 775. Tijuca. Rio de Janeiro. CEP 20.270-004. Entrance via Orthopaedics, 4th floor).

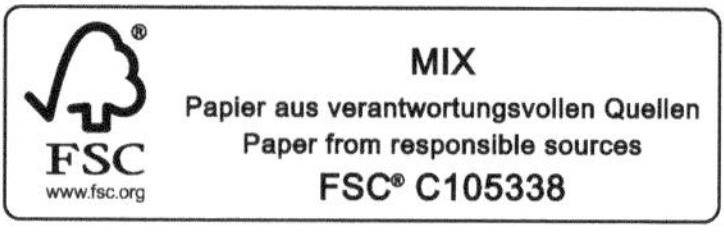

Printed by Books on Demand GmbH, Norderstedt / Germany